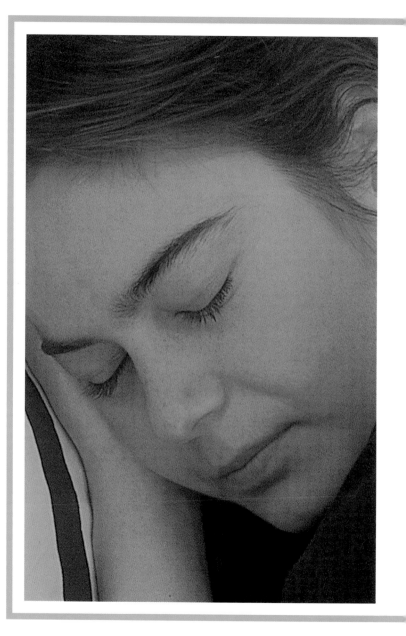

HELP
YOURSELF
to HEALTH

Sleep

*Practical ways to restore health
using complementary medicine*

PROF. EDZARD ERNST
MD, PH. D., FRCP (EDIN)

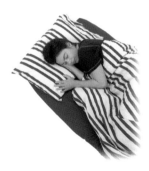

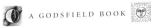

A GODSFIELD BOOK

Library of Congress Cataloging-in-Publication Data Available

10 9 8 7 6 5 4 3 2 1

Published in 1999 by Sterling Publishing Company, Inc.
387 Park Avenue South, New York, N.Y. 10016

DESIGNED FOR GODSFIELD PRESS BY
THE BRIDGEWATER BOOK COMPANY LTD

Picture research *Lynda Marshall*
Illustrations *Kevin Jones Associates and Michael Courtney*
Studio Photography *Zul Mukhida*

Distributed in Canada by Sterling Publishing
c/o Canadian Manda Group, One Atlantic Avenue, Suite 105
Toronto, Ontario, Canada M6K 3E7
Distributed in Australia by Capricorn Link (Australia) Pty Ltd
P O. Box 6651, Baulkham Hills, Business Centre, NSW 2153, Australia

Printed and bound in Hong Kong

ISBN 0-8069-3133-7

CONTENTS

INTRODUCTION

SLEEP IS OVERWHELMINGLY *important for all of us. For some it feels like lost time, while others are inspired by it. No other activity (yes, sleep is an activity) in our lives takes up more time – it has been estimated that we sleep on average for a total of 25 years of our entire life!*

Sleep has inspired poets, composers, and painters. It has also puzzled humankind for millennia. Researchers have studied different aspects of sleep with enthusiasm, rigor, and increasing success. Yet, at present, we still have more questions than answers relating to sleep.

Only about 20 percent of people living in industrialized countries have no sleep disturbances at all. About 25 to 35 percent suffer from severe sleep-related problems that require medical attention. The rest of us have minor, often recurrent sleep disturbances, for an average of at least five nights per month.

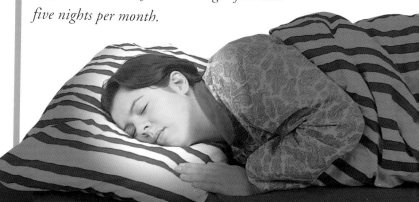

If you suffer from sleep-related problems you will, no doubt, have sought help, either from a doctor or elsewhere. In the United States, about 40 percent of the population presently use complementary therapies. In

ABOVE *Sleep is inspiration to artists and poets.*

Germany, this figure is as high as 65 percent. The vast array of remedies on offer may confuse you – you can always ask your physician about conventional medical treatments, but with complementary approaches, doctors often know little more than their patients.

The aim of this book is to guide you through the maze of these treatments. In order to offer you informed choices, the book will also outline some basic concepts of sleep-related problems, their causes and effects. The strengths and weaknesses of conventional treatments will also be mentioned, but the main part of the book is dedicated to complementary therapies

BELOW *Sleep is fundamental to our happiness and well-being.*

WHAT IS INSOMNIA?

Insomnia is defined as a lack of sleep, in quality or quantity. Women, older people, and those living alone tend to suffer the most from insomnia. Here we look at how and why people are afflicted by this complaint.

Various types of insomnia can be identified, chiefly by looking at the cause and severity of the problem. In addition, difficulties falling asleep can be differentiated from waking during the night.

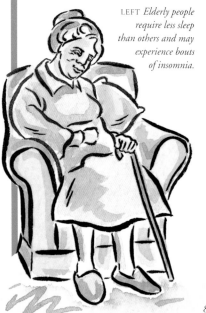

LEFT *Elderly people require less sleep than others and may experience bouts of insomnia.*

THE CAUSES OF INSOMNIA

There are four basic categories:

✧ Insomnia without apparent reason ("normal" insomnia), doctors call this "primary insomnia."

✧ Insomnia that is caused by other physical diseases.

✧ Insomnia due to mental disease.

✧ Insomnia due to external factors such as noise.

PRIMARY INSOMNIA

The most frequent form of insomnia is the one that has no apparent source or reason, the "normal" (or primary) insomnia. Strictly speaking, however, you can only be sure about this diagnosis once you have excluded the other categories listed above.

PHYSICAL DISEASES

A large list of physical diseases are associated with insomnia. Obviously, pain will cause sleep problems. Other conditions that often hinder sleep are the following:

- ◇ Congestive heart failure
- ◇ Chronic cough
- ◇ Hyperactive thyroid
- ◇ The menopause
- ◇ Drug addictions
- ◇ Asthma
- ◇ Prostate problems
- ◇ Several diseases of the brain or nervous system

BELOW *Other health problems may be the cause of insomnia. But for many there is no apparent reason for the inability to sleep.*

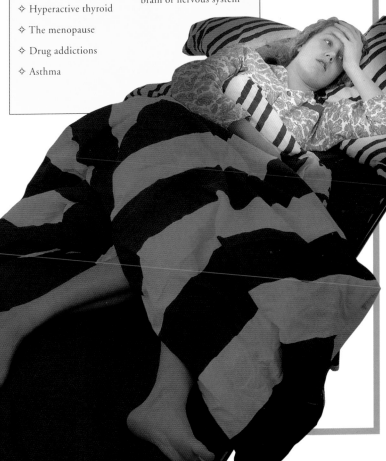

MENTAL DISEASES

Mental diseases, most prominently depression, are regularly linked with sleep problems. Here again, it is essential to treat the underlying condition (depression) rather than one of its symptoms (insomnia).

BELOW *A common cold could easily cause insomnia.*

EXTERNAL FACTORS

Finally, there is a long list of external factors that lead to sleep disturbances. These factors can be blatantly obvious, such as the noise level within the environment, too high temperatures in the bedroom, or an uncomfortable bed. Or they can result from far less obvious sources, including side effects from medication. Many drugs can cause sleep problems. They may not do this in all cases, some only in rare instances. Yet it is important to know of their potential to disrupt sleep.

OVERLAPPING CATEGORIES

It is clear that all classifications of insomnia are somewhat arbitrary. In each individual case there can be (and often is) a mixture of categories and causes. For instance, noise can be an obvious

DRUGS THAT MAY DISRUPT SLEEP

✧ *Amantadine*

✧ *Appetite suppressants*

✧ *Barbiturates*

✧ *Benzodiazepine*

✧ *Chloroquin*

✧ *L-tryptophane*

✧ *MAO inhibitors*

✧ *Neuroleptics*

✧ *Phenothiazine*

✧ *Piracetam*

✧ *Psychostimulants*

✧ *Scopolamine*

✧ *Thyroid hormones*

✧ *Tranquilizers*

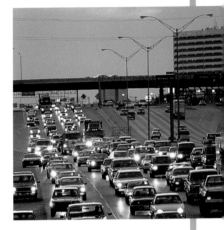

ABOVE *Noise pollution can come from all sorts of sources and may be difficult to overcome.*

CAUTION!

This list of drugs (above left) makes two important things quite clear. First, insomnia can be related to serious diseases. Therefore, it is essential that in all cases a correct diagnosis is made by a physician who has experience with insomnia. Second, if insomnia is caused by a specific disease, it is no good (even dangerous) to try to treat it with sleeping pills because in such cases only the adequate treatment of the underlying cause will bring success.

reason for bad sleep. But the same level of noise would not disturb a healthy person and might cause severe problems for someone suffering from depression or regular intervals of pain. In most sleep disturbance cases there is more than one single cause for the problem and one may amplify the other – physical discomfort, for example, can cause depression.

THE DURATION
OF INSOMNIA

Another way of classifying insomnia is by the severity of the problem:

- *Transient insomnia (just one or two nights of disturbed sleep).*
- *Short-term insomnia (no longer than three weeks).*
- *Chronic insomnia (longer than three weeks).*

Transient insomnia is experienced by every individual at some time or another. It has no real importance and certainly does not require treatment.

Short-term insomnia can be due to an acute underlying condition, e.g. pain or a cough. In other cases it may be the start of a chronic problem.

Chronic insomnia always requires medical attention but can be treated effectively. If you suffer from it you

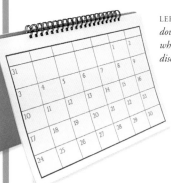

LEFT *Try to note down on a calender when your sleep disorder began.*

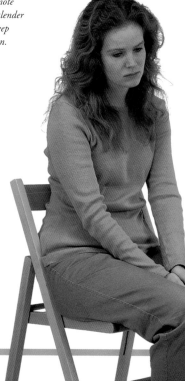

SLEEP LABORATORIES

Those suffering from chronic or complex sleep disorders may be referred to a sleep laboratory. These are found in most major hospitals and have been set up to monitor people's sleep patterns in order to diagnose a patient's disorder correctly.

should see your doctor and insist that your problem is adequately diagnosed; this may take patience and determination according to the response that you receive. Because insomnia may be a symptom of other problems, it may take some time to isolate and diagnose underlying causes. Only after a correct diagnosis can you begin to take informed choices about the best form of treatment.

CHRONIC INSOMNIA IS OFTEN RELATED TO

✧ Unhealthy living

✧ Not enough exercise

✧ Overworking

✧ Anxiety

✧ Stress

✧ Irregularity of lifestyle

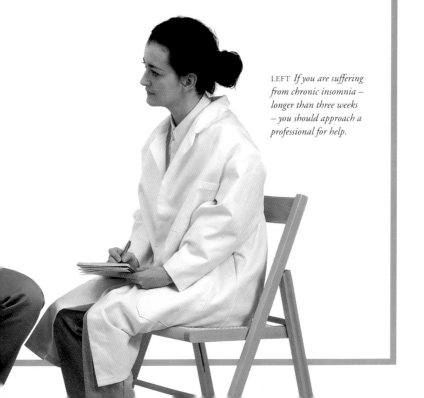

LEFT *If you are suffering from chronic insomnia – longer than three weeks – you should approach a professional for help.*

SLEEP DISTURBANCES FREQUENTLY HAVE MORE THAN ONE CAUSE

We all know how awful you can feel after a truly bad night's sleep. Even those with perfectly good sleep patterns can be affected by insomnia as part of everyday life. It is estimated that in the United States 100,000 traffic accidents (10,000 with a fatal outcome) are a direct result of sleep-deprivation problems.

It is possible to visualize a vicious circle where sleep problems, once started, can easily perpetuate themselves.

Sleep disorders can begin so easily, just a few hours lost because of a late night may result in sleepiness the next morning. This may worsen at work, especially if you are under pressure. You're exhausted, but when you finally get into bed you cannot sleep. The next day you are even more agitated,

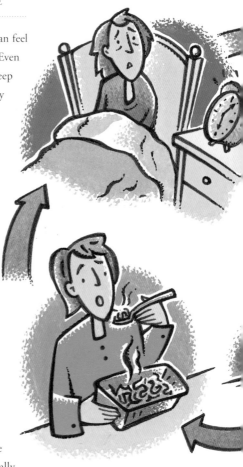

BELOW *An early start may be a shock to your system.*

ABOVE *There is too much to do and you leave eating dinner to the last thing.*

BELOW *Work can increase stress and anxiety.*

work seems even more demanding, there is less and less time to cook dinner and eat properly. Sometimes this kind of vicious circle can lead to serious conditions such as apnea – a temporary cessation of breathing which occurs during sleep. Apnea may not necessarily be linked to stress at work and home, but the condition is no doubt worsened by stress. Anyone suffering from this condition should seek medical treatment immediately.

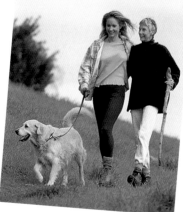

ABOVE *You simply can't get anywhere fast enough.*

ABOVE *Take a break from your normal routine.*

SPECIFIC SLEEP-RELATED PROBLEMS

In addition to the insomnia types mentioned in the previous pages, there are very specific problems that occur predominantly at night and regularly go with sleep disturbances.

SNORING

Snoring is clearly a problem for the person who has to listen to it. What is less well known is that it also harms the snorer. Men are affected more often than women, so are overweight individuals and smokers. There is some evidence to suggest that snorers are more at greater risk of cardiovascular disease than non snorers.

Snoring is also often associated with sleep apnea. People with this condition stop breathing at more or less regular intervals. The pause can be longer than one minute. To the observer, these intervals of absolute silence are therefore clearly recognizable. Sleep apnea is a serious and treatable problem and needs urgent expert medical attention. Because the person afflicted with it breathes less, his or

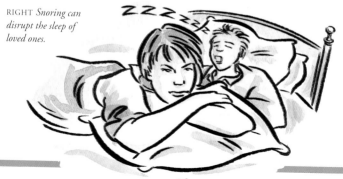

RIGHT *Snoring can disrupt the sleep of loved ones.*

TREATING THE PROBLEM

✧ There are several ways to treat snoring. If applicable, reducing weight and giving up smoking are the two obvious first steps.

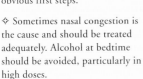

✧ Sometimes nasal congestion is the cause and should be treated adequately. Alcohol at bedtime should be avoided, particularly in high doses.

✧ Vocal exercises that tone the soft palate are a promising approach – snoring is mostly caused by too much relaxation in this area.

LEFT *Snoring can be a result of habits such as smoking.*

✧ Avoidance of sleeping on the back (try attaching a tennis ball to the back of your pajama top) may also put an end to your snoring.

✧ For extreme and desperate cases, a doctor might even suggest surgery to the palate.

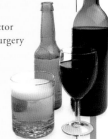

RIGHT *Alcohol at bedtime may not be conducive to sleep.*

her blood runs dangerously low in oxygen, which can cause severe problems in tissue supply to organs such as the brain or the heart. Sufferers will usually have poor-quality sleep. The result would be episodes of extreme tiredness during the day time.

RESTLESS LEG SYNDROME

This condition is characterized by the compulsive movement of legs while lying in bed. This prevents sleep for those directly afflicted by it and makes it difficult for the partner who shares a bed as well. Restless leg syndrome can be caused by diseases such as diabetes, renal failure, polyneuropathy, or anemia. Therefore, it is essential that you see your doctor when you suffer from this condition. There are several treatment options that may bring relief to those who suffer from this syndrome. But most important, the underlying condition (if any) needs to be diagnosed and treated.

CRAMPS

Many people suffer from painful leg cramps that wake them at night. Such cramps can have specific causes (e.g. an imbalance of electrolytes in your blood), which are treatable once correctly diagnosed. Therefore, it is important to see your doctor if you suffer from nocturnal leg cramps. In most cases, however, cramps have no identifiable cause – physicians would then speak of idiopathic cramps. In such cases a number of therapeutic options exist.

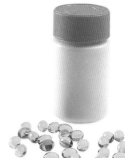

LEFT *A dose of vitamin E will reduce the regularity of cramp.*

THERAPIES FOR CRAMP

✧ Stretching exercise.

✧ Oral medication with quinine (unfortunately not free of risk).

✧ Vitamin E.

✧ Homeopathic cuprum – many homeopaths insist that this works but there is, as yet, no hard evidence to prove it.

LEFT *To relieve pain from cramps in your legs try to keep still and gently stretch.*

RAISE AND STRETCH LEG

STRETCH OUT FOOT

There are other, more readily available remedies for cramp sufferers: bananas give carbohydrate energy and provide a dose of potassium, which prevents cramps. Night cramps can also be relieved by eating a few nuts or seeds, some extra-virgin olive oil, or an avocado each day to provide extra vitamin E, which aids circulation. You may also find that a massage with lavender oil before you go to sleep will make all the difference. Lavender is used by aromatherapists to soothe and relax. Herbalists may recommend "Cramp Bark Ointment" for the same purpose.

TEETH GRINDING

People who grind their teeth while asleep do not usually sleep badly – but their spouses might be unable to sleep because of it. The reason for teeth grinding is unknown, although it has been suggested that teeth grinding is linked to stress and anxiety. Wearing a simple device in the mouth will stop the problem and prevent any damage to the teeth.

PANIC ATTACKS

Panic attacks at night are uncontrollable episodes of fear during waking. They can be brought on by some medications or by anxiety, but more often they are linked to depression. If panic attacks become a regular problem, consult you doctor.

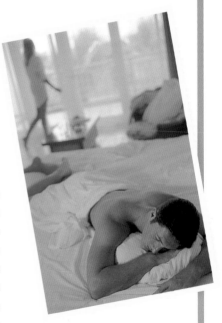

ABOVE *Teeth grinding is often more disturbing for the sufferer's partner.*

JET LAG

Long-haul flights through time zones tend to upset the inner clock. The problem is more pronounced when flying from west to east. When we suffer from jet lag, our bodies tell us to sleep when we cannot (e.g. because we have business to conduct) and it prevents us from sleeping when we try to sleep at night. The result is a lack of concentration and appetite, headaches, tiredness, irritability, etc.

ABOVE *A flight across different time zones causes the phenomenon of jetlag.*

BELOW *In order to combat jet lag, try to stick to your normal routine.*

There are several simple tips that you can follow to beat the problem:

✧

Adopt the timetable of your destination as you embark on your journey; try not to think about what time it is at home.

✧

Insist on regular physical exercise.

RIGHT *If you are already fit and healthy you are less likely to suffer from jet lag.*

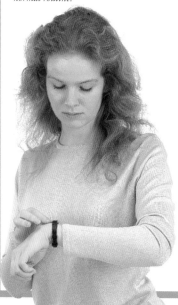

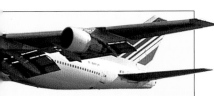

NIGHTMARES

Nightmares are frightening dreams that are experienced by most of us at some stage. They are not normally associated with insomnia. If nightmares are a regular occurrence, consult your doctor and consider seeing a psychologist.

Try to get some sleep during the flight.

❖

Start your journey well rested.

❖

Avoid alcohol, tea, coffee, and nicotine, both en route and during the period when jet lag might hit you.

❖

Try a short-acting sleeping pill (see page 33) to sleep the night through at your destination or on a night flight.

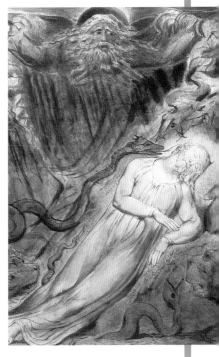

ABOVE *Our imaginations can conjure up terrifying night images.*

ESSENTIAL FACTS ABOUT SLEEP

Sleep is an essential element of our lives; we cannot choose not to sleep. If we have too little sleep, all sorts of problems are likely to arise.

About 50 percent of all accidents are caused by lack of quality sleep. With fatal accidents this figure could even be higher. If it continues for long periods of time, insomnia inevitably causes other health problems. Generally speaking, people who sleep well are healthier and live longer than those who do not. They are also more productive and efficient. The first thing that we notice when we have slept badly is that our mood is down. Therefore, a good night's sleep also improves people's sense of well-being and produces happier, more stable individuals.

It is surprisingly difficult to say exactly why we need sleep or even to define what sleep is. Sleep is not the

BELOW *Sleep deprivation may cause concentration loss – a danger to others as well as yourself.*

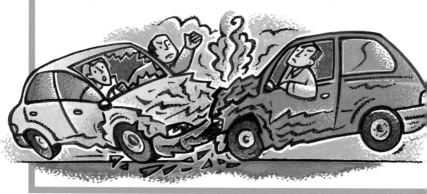

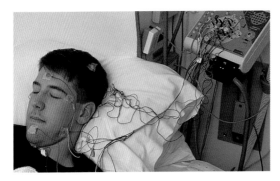

LEFT *Researchers are able to monitor sleep patterns using electrodes.*

same as resting or doing nothing. Scientifically speaking, sleep is a state of reduced consciousness with loss of responsiveness to the environment, partial loss of mental function, and total loss of short-term memory.

STATES OF SLEEP

Researchers distinguish two distinct states of sleep. One is characterized by rapid eye movements and is therefore called REM sleep. The other has no rapid eye movements and is aptly termed NREM sleep. Each normal night's sleep comprises four or five cycles of alternating NREM and REM sleep. Each cycle lasts for 90–120 minutes.

QUIET PHASE

NREM sleep is the quiet phase in which the brain is relatively inactive. This is not to say that the body as a whole is inactive. Most body systems are working hard during NREM sleep: some produce hormones, others proteins; obviously all the essential functions such as breathing, blood circulation, and digestion carry on. NREM sleep goes through a succession of four stages. The deepness of sleep increases from stage one to four. Each stage is characterized by typical brain activity that can be measured in a sleep laboratory by attaching electrical wires to the skull. NREM sleep rejuvenates us.

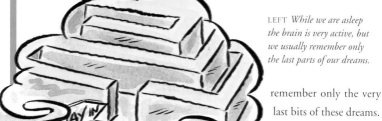

LEFT *While we are asleep the brain is very active, but we usually remember only the last parts of our dreams.*

remember only the very last bits of these dreams.

Each episode of REM sleep lasts for about a half hour. The hallmark of REM sleep is an active brain and a totally dissociated, inactive, and relaxed body. At this stage, the brain abandons part of its usual

DREAM MODE

After about 90 minutes of NREM sleep, REM sleep normally starts. The rapid eye movements that give it its name are a reflection of the high level of brain activity. It is during this period that we dream. We usually

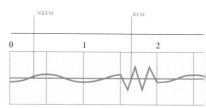

control over bodily functions. There is, for instance, no longer a tight control over body temperature which fluctuates. Also, the heartbeat and breathing patterns become erratic. As most muscles are totally relaxed, breathing is performed not, as usual, with the assistance of the muscles of the rib cage but only through the contractions of the diaphragm.

The function of REM sleep is not well understood. Some experts think it is important in terms of memory and learning.

AN AVERAGE NIGHT

During an average night, our sleep would be composed of roughly the following phases: fetuses spend most of their time in REM sleep; new-born babies spend about half their time sleeping; and the graph below shows the sleep pattern of an average adult.

BELOW *During the night we will experience different phases of sleep – on average, one and a half hours of NREM sleep will alternate with 30 minutes REM.*

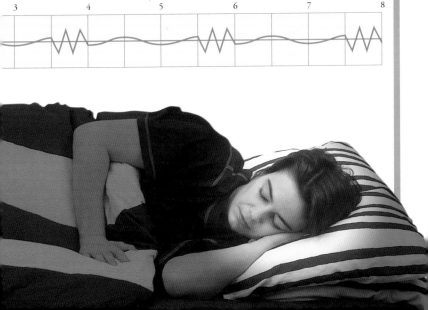

HOURS					
3	4	5	6	7	8

HOW MUCH IS ENOUGH?

Some people need little sleep, others require much more. It is problematic therefore to give guidelines, but it is possible to provide averages. Generally speaking, we need less sleep as we grow older.

SLEEP REQUIREMENTS

- *Babies need between 14 and 16 hours per 24 hours.*
- *Children between 5 and 15 years need about 9 hours.*

- *Adolescents need about 11 hours.*
- *Adults need about 8 hours.*
- *Elderly people need about 6 hours.*

BELOW *Our need for sleep is often dictated by age.*

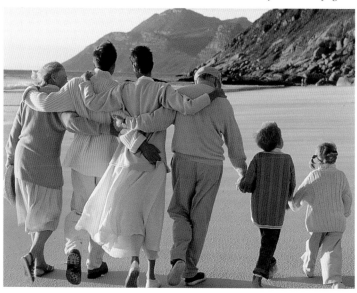

IDENTIFYING A PROBLEM

Waking up at night is normal. It becomes a problem only if you cannot fall swiftly back to sleep. The waking time during the night increases with age.

Many think they have a sleep problem while, in fact, everything is quite normal. Some people do not realize that as little as five hours may be quite sufficient for their own personal needs.

Others underestimate the time that they have actually slept – the time you spend trying to go to sleep is memorized (and often seems to last forever), while the time during which you sleep, of course, is not committed to memory. Therefore, it can be difficult to ascertain whether or not a given individual has a problem.

If the answer is yes to the majority of the questions in the box, then you should see your doctor and discuss the possibility of a sleep-related problem. If it proves impossible to establish the diagnosis otherwise, small devices are now available that are worn almost like a wristwatch and detect body movements – this will then give you or your doctor a more reliable indication as to how much you really sleep.

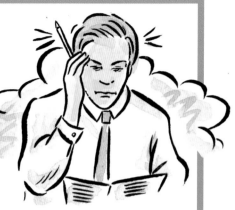

ABOVE *A physician may not be able to make his diagnosis immediately.*

DO YOU HAVE INSOMNIA?

Answering the questions below may help in determining whether you have a sleep problem:

✧ Do you regularly wake up in the morning feeling groggy?

✧ Do you regularly feel like dozing off during the day?

✧ Do you often find it hard to concentrate?

✧ Do you often have problems with your memory?

AGGRAVATING FACTORS

There are several factors that are rarely the sole cause for insomnia but are very often a contributing factor that make things worse once insomnia has become a problem.

ALCOHOL

Many people think that alcohol enhances sleep. It is possible that a "night cap" can have this effect by reducing anxiety. But certainly larger quantities of alcohol are likely to make you wake up during the night and reduce your quality of sleep. Pharmacologically speaking, alcohol is a powerful and long-acting stimulant; therefore, its detrimental effect on sleep does not come as a surprise.

SMOKING

Nicotine is also a stimulant and can ruin your sleep. Smoking insomniacs should seriously consider kicking the habit. The chances are that they will find, once they have gone through the immediate period of withdrawal, their sleep much improved. Since smoking is seriously damaging to your health in many other ways, this is most certainly worth a try.

OTHER STIMULANTS

What goes for alcohol and cigarettes goes for virtually all stimulants. Tea and coffee are classic examples; so are medications that pep you up, including some herbal remedies, e.g. Ginseng or Ephedra.

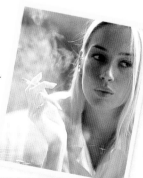

RIGHT
Smoking is now especially common among younger women. It may worsen insomnia.

WHAT TO AVOID

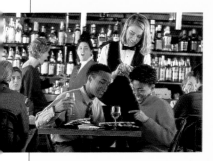

LEFT *Overindulgence can affect your sleep.*

Stimulants such as alcohol and cigarette smoke and a series of late nights may add further disruption to your sleep patterns. Over-indulgence and late nights should be avoided if you are concerned about the quality of your sleep.

Caffeine is also an obvious hindrance to sleep, although it can improve mental performance. It is found mainly in coffee and tea, but is also present in chocolate, some fizzy drinks, and some cold and pain relief tablets.

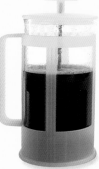
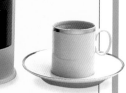

LEFT *Caffeine may affect your ability to sleep.*

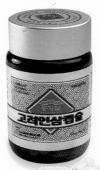

LEFT *Natural stimulants such as Ginseng can be used to treat lethargy as well as insomnia.*

Ginseng, Ephedra, Guavana are all natural stimulants that you can buy over the counter. They are taken by those who want to increase their performance and energy levels. Ginseng is a particularly valuable herb which treats lethargy but also has a proven calming affect. It is used to treat palpitations, anxiety and restlessness as well as insomnia.

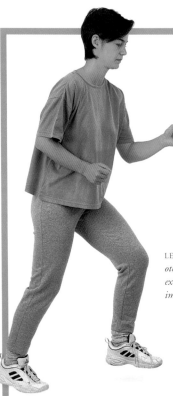

STRESS AND ANXIETY

Many of us lead lifestyles that not only provide too little exercise but far too much stress, worry, and anxiety. This, in turn, can significantly contribute to sleep problems. It is important to be able to "switch-off" occasionally.

LEFT *Running, or other forms of exercise, may improve your sleep.*

BELOW *Insomniacs are often unable to switch off and stop thinking.*

LACK OF EXERCISE

It seems quite logical that a lack of physical exertion would aggravate sleep problems. Even if your job gives you little occasion, you should find yourself a sport or hobby that is physically challenging. The effect on sleep can be quite dramatic (see pages 58–59).

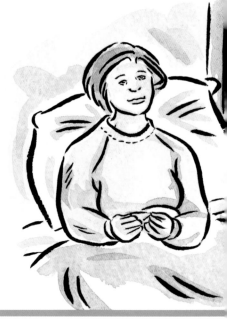

MEDICINES

Prescribed drugs can contribute to sleep disturbances (see page 11). If you are taking such medications, it is important to realize that your sleep problem might stem partly from this. Discuss these matters with your physician – he or she might reduce the dosage or prescribe a different drug that affects you less.

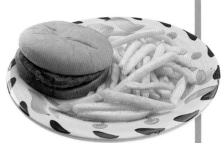

ABOVE *Avoid eating meals packed with carbohydrates close to bedtime.*

FOOD

Heavy meals, eaten late in the evening, are an important and common contributor to sleep problems. In particular, animal fat and too large meals may be the culprit. It might be worth taking note of which foodstuffs have what effect on your sleep – this may be different from person to person. Generally speaking it is advisable, particularly for elderly people, to eat light and early (at least two hours before bedtime) to enhance sleep in the hours to follow.

CONVENTIONAL TREATMENTS

This book is not about conventional treatments of insomnia. However, to make informed choices, it is necessary to mention briefly all the major options. As you will see, some types of treatment can be looked upon as either mainstream or complementary, depending which way you look at them.

Generally speaking, with insomnia, as with most other medical conditions, the earlier you start treatment the better. As a rule, a sufferer needs medical attention if he or she:

● *Feels lack of regeneration through sleep.*
● *Is becoming increasingly concerned about bad sleep and its consequences.*
● *Is finding that daytime activities are being limited as a result of sleep deprivation.*

The main aims of any treatment, regardless of whether conventional or complementary, are to eliminate causes and aggravation factors and to restore sleep quality and quantity.

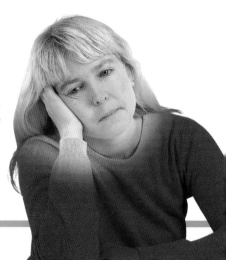

RIGHT *The main aim in seeking treatment is to restore sleep.*

SLEEPING PILLS

It has been estimated that 40 million Americans suffer from sleep-related problems. The medical profession is badly equipped to deal with such an endemic; doctors learn very little about sleeping disorders in basic training. As a result, writing a prescription for a sleeping pill is almost a reflex response. Yet this is not necessarily an adequate solution. In many cases pills can make the problem worse.

CAUTION!

It is clear that sleeping pills should be handled with the utmost caution. Disregard of this general rule has ruined thousands of lives.

Here are some simple rules for dealing with sleeping pills:

View sleeping pills only as a temporary solution; do not use them for more than two weeks.

❖

Be aware that they can be addictive. In order to achieve a constant effect, higher and higher doses are required.

❖

Note that when discontinuing sleeping pills, sleep can temporarily be worse than before.

❖

Be aware that long-term use can cause severe organ damage (e.g. kidneys, nerve fibers)

❖

Note that sometimes sleeping pills can hinder sleep rather than enhance it

❖

Note that sleeping pills do not promote vital REM sleep

IMPORTANT FEATURES OF DIFFERENT TYPES OF SLEEPING PILLS

Name or category of drug	Sleep latency	Sleep time	Sleep quality	Other quality
Tricyclic antidepressants	↓	?	?	potential for serious side-effects, low abuse potential
Trazodone	↓	↑	—	potential for side-effects
Barbiturates	↓	↑	?	addictive, overdose can be lethal
Bendodiaepaines	↓	↑	↑	very commonly used, relatively safe
Chloral hydrate	↓	↑	?	should not be taken by people with liver, kidney, or heart problems, or those who are on warfarin or oral anti-diabetic medication
Zaleplon	↓	↑	?	new drug with promising characteristics
Zolpidem	↓	↑	↑	can also decrease the frequency of night-time awakenings
Zopicolone	↓	↑	↑	decreases night-time awakenings

KEY　↓ = DECREASE　? = NOT KNOWN　— = NO EFFECT　↑ = INCREASE

NON-DRUG THERAPIES

Many healthcare professionals have fully realized the numerous disadvantages of chemical sleeping pills. Depending on their background, they therefore recommend the following:

- *Psychological treatments, e.g. counseling, cognitive therapy, behavioral therapy.*
- *Relaxation therapies.*
- *Sleep restriction.*
- *Psychotherapy.*

All of these approaches may be useful either by themselves or in combination. Psychological approaches tend to be popular since they do not involve tablets, do appear to make sense, and provide time, attention, and reassurance. These methods are also called "talking treatments." Unfortunately, trained personnel may not always be available, so demand often outstrips the supply. These therapies are time consuming and therefore expensive.

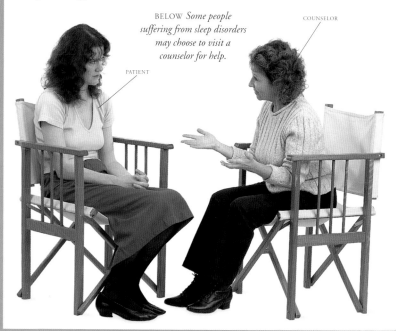

BELOW *Some people suffering from sleep disorders may choose to visit a counselor for help.*

COUNSELOR

PATIENT

COUNSELING

Counseling can be viewed as an extension and refinement of everyday ways of helping suffering individuals.

In addition to providing supportive therapy on a one-to-one basis, counseling reviews problems and aggravating factors. The therapist may encourage the patient to set goals and make changes to help to solve problems. This may involve keeping a diary of sleep and emotional patterns.

As well as providing information and advice about insomnia, the counselor can encourage the expression of emotion and the sharing of feelings. Step-by-step problem-solving strategies can be taught and implemented.

COGNITIVE BEHAVIOR THERAPY (CBT)

CBT aims to change patterns of thinking and behavior that interfere with sleep. CBT is also used to treat depression, which may be the cause of sleep problems. It focuses on teaching people how to control their thoughts, emotions, and behaviors. Various types of negative thinking – that keep the mind full of fears and anxieties –

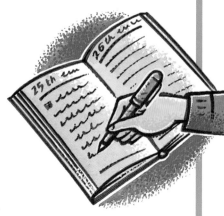

BELOW *A counselor may encourage his or her patients to keep a diary recording their sleep patterns.*

may perpetuate or aggravate the sleep problem. By working closely with a clinical psychologist, ways of challenging and changing these thought patterns can be developed.

CBT usually consists of 6- to 20-hour-long sessions taking place at weekly intervals. Diaries of daily thoughts and activities are usually kept, and often "homework" exercises are given in addition. Considerable commitment is therefore necessary from the patient – this therapy is really for those who are determined to break their habit of night worrying.

COMPLEMENTARY THERAPIES

The blanket term "complementary therapies" covers a wide variety of approaches and techniques. The following section of this book aims to guide you through the bewildering choice of treatments available, by describing what has been shown scientifically to work for insomnia and suggesting what holds promise.

Surveys in the United States, the UK, Australia, and Germany have shown that between 40 and 65 percent of the general population have tried complementary therapies in the last year. Insomnia is one of the most frequent reasons for trying complementary therapies. The roots for this growing popularity include a need to take control over one's own health problems, a disillusionment with orthodox medical approaches, a growing willingness to experiment with new methods, the need for time and attention from a caring therapist, and a desire for treatments that are seen to be more "natural" and are therefore thought to be free from unwanted side effects. This last point is unfortunately a misconception for, as will be expanded upon later, treatments using "natural" products and methods are not necessarily risk free.

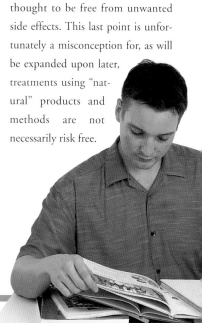

WHICH TREATMENT?

How can you decide where to start when faced with the perplexing array of choices? If you look at books on complementary medicine – and there are certainly plenty of them available – all sorts of therapies are proposed as a treatment for insomnia.

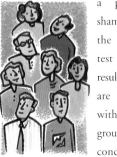

ABOVE *In a randomized controlled trial, only one group is given the treatment under investigation.*

But how is it possible to find out if any of these really work, or if they involve unexpected hazards? The most reliable method for establishing whether or not a treatment works is known as the randomized controlled trial. This term describes a surprisingly simple idea. A group of insomnia sufferers is divided through random allocation into two equal subgroups. Then they receive the treatment under investigation (group A) or another intervention (group B, the control group). This can be an existing treatment that has already been shown to work, no treatment at all, or a placebo or sham therapy. At the end of the test period, the results of group A are compared with those of group B to give a conclusion. The trial makes it possible to test whether the treatment under investigation works better than that given to the control group.

EARLY DAYS

The amount of research carried out on complementary therapies in the treatment of insomnia is so far fairly limited. But studies are ongoing. This means that the jury is still out for most of these therapies, and more good-quality research needs to be funded and carried out.

LEFT *Many people may begin their inquiries into self-help by reading about the subject.*

MELATONIN

Melatonin might well be seen as conventional by some people and as complementary by others. Since it is sold mostly through health food stores in the United States, the latter category seems more appropriate.

Melatonin is a hormone that is naturally produced in the brain. One of its functions is to control the day–night rhythm of our "inner clock." The discovery that melatonin levels are 10–50 fold higher one to two hours before bedtime tempted researchers to find out whether oral administration of this substance in the form of tablets would induce sleep.

ABOVE *The discovery of melatonin has led to a therapy for sufferers of insomnia. Melatonin is a natural hormone that increases the time spent asleep.*

DOES IT HELP?

Most of the clinical trials in fact suggest that melatonin decreases the time between going to bed and falling asleep and increases the total sleep time. In addition, some studies suggest that it also improves the quality of sleep. There are, however, several caveats. First, most studies were conducted on healthy people, and the few on insomniacs are contradictory. Second, large doses may be required – trials using 1 or 5mg showed no result, other studies using 75mg demonstrated a positive effect.

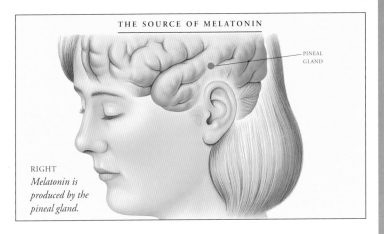

THE SOURCE OF MELATONIN

PINEAL GLAND

RIGHT
*Melatonin is
produced by the
pineal gland.*

THE QUESTION
OF SIDE EFFECTS

Some people are concerned about the side effects melatonin may have on users. Much uncertainty still exists concerning this point. In the trials mentioned above, few side effects were noted, but to be sure we need more data. In rare cases, people have experienced fatigue (obviously), headache, dizziness, and increased irritability after taking melatonin.

The list on the right shows us that it may be wise to err on the safe side and use melatonin, if at all, with great caution.

MELATONIN SHOULD NOT BE TAKEN BY PEOPLE WHO:

✧
Have problems with their immune system.
✧
Have diseases of the lymph system.
✧
Take immuno-suppressants.
✧
Take cortcosteroids.
✧
Are trying to become, or are, pregnant.
✧
Are breast-feeding.
✧
Have vascular disorders.
✧
Suffer from depression.

HERBAL TREATMENTS

Since prehistoric times plants have provided medicines. Each culture has developed its own tradition of herbal medicine. Today medicine relies largely on synthetic drugs. However, it should not be forgotten that many valuable drugs were originally (and many still are) derived from plants.

Among the branches of herbal medicine are traditional Chinese medicine, Indian Ayurvedic medicine, Japanese Kampo medicine, and Western herbalism. Herbal extracts normally contain many active substances. Often it is not known which chemicals are responsible for the medicinal effects. It is rarely understood by exactly what mechanism the extract works.

RIGHT *Chinese doctors have been prescribing herbal remedies, in the form of tea and soup, for millennia.*

SAFETY POINTS

The fact that plants occur naturally does not necessarily mean that they are entirely safe. Some of the most deadly poisons are plant products! The only difference between a safe drug and a poison is really the dose.

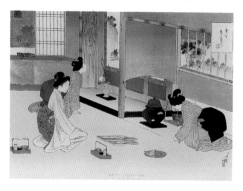

Even if a plant has a long history of use, it is possible that it may have side effects that are slow to develop or not very obvious so they have been overlooked in the past. As a general rule, herbal treatments are contraindicated during pregnancy or lactation unless there is convincing evidence to the contrary.

QUALITY CONTROL

The misidentification of the relevant plant species, or the intentional or accidental adulteration of the herbal remedy with toxic materials or conventional drugs, has also been a problem in the past. The content of a herbal remedy is likely to vary according to the source of the plant, the parts of the plant used, and the extraction procedure. Therefore, it is important that adequate quality control takes place. The best way you can assure quality is to buy from a reputable firm.

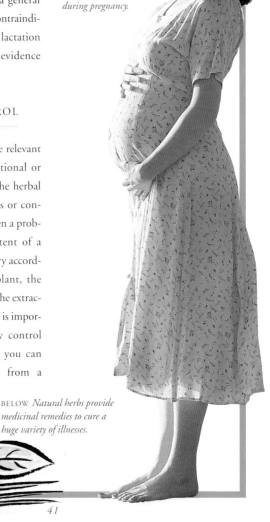

RIGHT *Herbal remedies are not recommended during pregnancy.*

BELOW *Natural herbs provide medicinal remedies to cure a huge variety of illnesses.*

VALERIAN

Valeriana officinalis is one of about 250 valerian species. It is a perennial plant, 20–60in (50–150cm) in height, which grows in Europe and Asia.

QUALITIES

Only its root is employed for medicinal purposes. A minimum of 2g dried herb is used to yield a single dose of about 400mg. The dried root contains 0.3–0.8 percent volatile oil.

More than 100 constituents have been identified, and it is still unknown which is the active principal. Studies in animals have shown that valerenic acid has sedative and anticonvulsant activity. Other investigations have demonstrated that valerian extracts increase the concentration of a neurotransmitter (GABA) that plays a role in stress and anxiety. Thus the relaxing effects of valerian are biologically plausible.

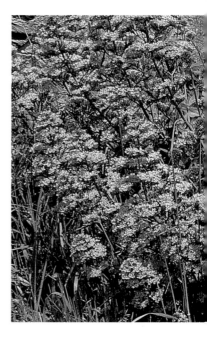

DOSAGE

The adequate dose of valerian is 400–600mg two hours before bedtime. It is important to realize that this regimen has to be followed for several weeks for the full benefit of the remedy to appear. For this reason, valerian is no ideal substitute for sleeping pills with immediate effects, but is most suited for medium-term treatment.

There are no reports about dependence. If you take other sleeping pills at the same time, the effects will add up – so be cautious. Valerian does not seem to interact with alcohol, as several other hypnotic medications do.

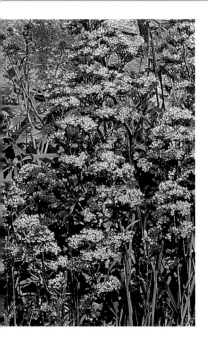

LEFT *Valerian (meaning "to be in health") has been used for centuries to relieve insomnia.*

that have been implicated in causing more severe problems. Mexican and Indian valerian contain relatively high concentrations of valepotriates. These varieties should therefore be avoided.

CLINICAL STUDIES

Tests show that with 400–1200mg valerian extract per day, given for 1 to 30 days, an improvement in the following symptoms can be expected:

❖

Behavioral disturbances

❖

Difficulty falling asleep

❖

Early waking

❖

Frequency of waking

❖

Inner tension

❖

Mood

❖

Nighttime motor activity

❖

Restlessness

❖

Sleep latency

❖

Sleep quality

SIDE EFFECTS

The clinical trials and other similar investigations also suggest that valerian is safe. With sleeping pills, one often encounters a loss of vigilance the day after taking them. This does not seem to be a problem with valerian. Mild side effects such as headaches, grogginess, and gastrointestinal complaints have been reported, but only occasionally. Good valerian extracts contain only traces of valepotriates

HOPS

....

In Europe, hops (*humulus lupulus*) were traditionally used as a diuretic, tonic, and bitter, but when it came to public attention that hop-pickers were often tired, this led to investigations into the plant's sedative properties.

QUALITIES

For medicinal purposes, hops strobiles are used. They contain the two chemicals, humulone and lupulone, that have sedative effects in test animals. Several studies in human patients suggest that hops extracts enhance sleep.

However, too few rigorous clinical trials have so far been performed to make final judgments.

DOSAGE

The recommended dose is 0.5g of the dried herb about two hours before bedtime.

SIDE EFFECTS

There are no reports about side effects other than rare cases of hops allergy. The sedative effects may be made stronger by concomitant hypnotic medication or alcohol. Hops may relax the uterus (particularly in high doses); therefore, there is a specific reason to avoid it during pregnancy.

STROBILE – SCALY FEMALE FLOWER

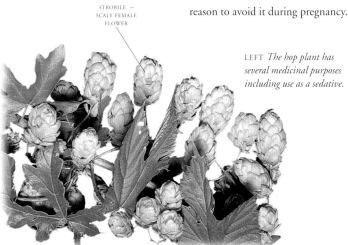

LEFT *The hop plant has several medicinal purposes including use as a sedative.*

LEMON BALM

Pills and teas of lemon balm are traditionally used to enhance sleep. However, there are no conclusive clinical trials to support its effectiveness.

QUALITIES

The leaves of lemon balm (*melissa officinalis*) contain at least 0.05 percent of volatile oil with its main constituents citronella, geranial, neral and phenol carboxylic acid including rosemarinic acid. An interesting new development is the demonstration of antiviral effects of lemon balm. A lemon balm cream against herpes labialis (a viral infection) is already on the market.

ABOVE *Use a pestle and mortar to crush fresh herbs.*

DOSAGE

The recommended dose is 1.5–4.5g of dried leaves about two hours before bedtime. Lemon balm can also be added fresh to salads and sauces.

SIDE EFFECTS

No known side effects of lemon balm are on record.

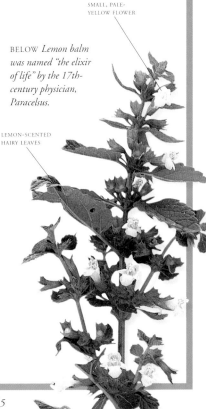

SMALL, PALE-YELLOW FLOWER

BELOW *Lemon balm was named "the elixir of life" by the 17th-century physician, Paracelsus.*

LEMON-SCENTED HAIRY LEAVES

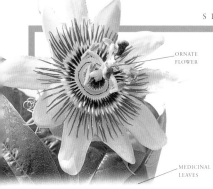

ORNATE
FLOWER

MEDICINAL
LEAVES

ABOVE *Passionflower leaves,
served as a tea, promote sleep.*

PASSIONFLOWER

A tropical climbing vine, passionflower (*passiflora incarnata*), native to the southern United States, has been traditionally used for reducing anxiety and relieving sleep problems.

QUALITIES

Its main constituents are flavonoids, coumarin and umbeliferone. Its pharmacological effect had been assumed to be due to harmala alkaloids but more recent research has cast some doubt on this notion. Passionflower extracts exhibit sedative effects on animals, but there have been no controlled clinical trials on humans.

RIGHT *Lavender flowers
should be harvested and dried.*

DOSAGE

The recommended dose is 4–8g two hours before bedtime.

SIDE EFFECTS

No side effects have been reported.

LAVENDER

The dried flowers of lavender (*Lavandula angustifolia*), gathered just before they open, are used for medicinal purposes. The shrub is indigenous in the Mediterranean.

QUALITIES

They contain at least 1.5 percent volatile oil with its main constituents linalyl acetate, linalool, camphor, beta-ocimene, and cineole. Animal experiments have shown the sedative action of lavender oil. There are few

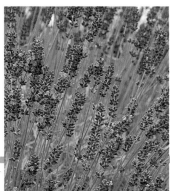

studies on human patients; these relate mostly to its use in aromatherapy (see pages 72–73).

DOSAGE

The recommended dose is 1–2 teaspoons of dried herb per cup as a tea, or 1–4 drops of lavender oil on a sugar cube, or 100g of dried flowers added to the bathwater for external use.

SIDE EFFECTS

Lavender has no known side effects.

ST. JOHN'S WORT

A herbaceous perennial, St. John's Wort (*Hypericum perforatum*) grows in Europe, Asia, and Africa.

QUALITIES

Recent research shows that it is effective as an antidepressant and in treating insomnia. The results of about 20 rigorous trials have been published and show that St. John's Wort helps to reduce the symptoms of insomnia during mild to moderate depression and that it is as effective as conventional antidepressants.

DOSAGE

2 to 4g herb daily or equivalents (0.5 to 3.0mg total hypericin daily).

SIDE EFFECTS

The most common unwanted effects reported with St. John's Wort are nausea, stomach ache, skin rashes, itching, and tiredness. These prob-

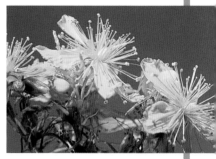

ABOVE *The yellow flowers of St. John's Wort.*

lems tend to be mild and to occur for only about 2 to 3 percent of people. There is a potential risk that the skin becomes hypersensitive to sunlight. This is highly unlikely to occur at the recommended doses. The trials mentioned above demonstrate that the frequency and severity of side effects of St. John's Wort are less than those of conventional antidepressants.

KAVA KAVA

The natives of Polynesia, Melanesia, and Micronesia have traditionally used the kava kava shrub (*piper methysticum*) to make a ceremonial drink with calming and relaxing effects. This led to the development of kava kava as an anxiolytic (anxiety-relieving) herbal remedy. Today the roots are dried and extracted for a liquid that is high in kavapyrones. In as much as sleep may be impeded by anxiety, kava kava extracts would also enhance sleep.

KAVA KAVA CLINICAL TRIALS

With dosages ranging from 30-210mg kavapyrones per day, improvements could be noted in the following complaints:

- Anxiety
- Climacteric symptoms
- Depression
- Mood

HERBAL TEAS

Several national pharmacopeias list herbal sedative tea preparations. Such teas are made with one tablespoon of the herbal mixture per cup. Pour boiling water over it, cover and steep for 10 minutes. Drink one cup 2–3 times per day, particularly 2–3 hours before going to bed. Opposite are standard prescriptions for various sedative tea preparations, which can be made up by a pharmacist.

USING KAVA KAVA

Side effects of kava kava are mild, transient, and rare. Only about 2 percent of patients are affected. Gastrointestinal symptoms, allergies, headache, and dizziness are the most frequent complaints. The recommended dose is 60–120mg kavapyrones per day for no more than three months. There is no reason to fear dependency.

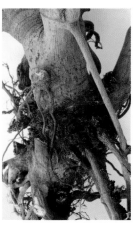

LEFT *The roots of the kava kava shrub are dried for use.*

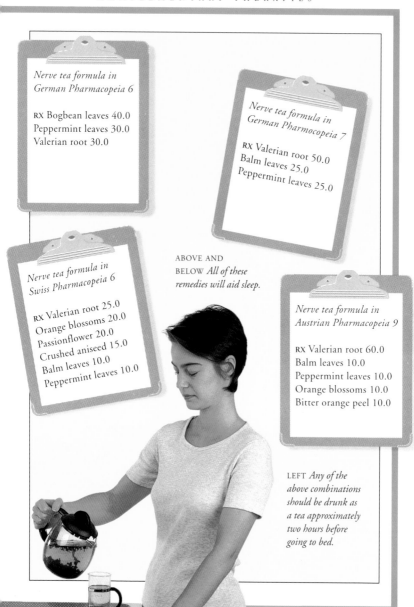

Nerve tea formula in German Pharmacopeia 6

RX Bogbean leaves 40.0
Peppermint leaves 30.0
Valerian root 30.0

Nerve tea formula in German Pharmocopeia 7

RX Valerian root 50.0
Balm leaves 25.0
Peppermint leaves 25.0

Nerve tea formula in Swiss Pharmacopeia 6

RX Valerian root 25.0
Orange blossoms 20.0
Passionflower 20.0
Crushed aniseed 15.0
Balm leaves 10.0
Peppermint leaves 10.0

ABOVE AND BELOW *All of these remedies will aid sleep.*

Nerve tea formula in Austrian Pharmacopeia 9

RX Valerian root 60.0
Balm leaves 10.0
Peppermint leaves 10.0
Orange blossoms 10.0
Bitter orange peel 10.0

LEFT *Any of the above combinations should be drunk as a tea approximately two hours before going to bed.*

HOMEOPATHY

Homeopathy was developed by the German doctor Samuel Hahnemann in the late 18th century. It is based on the principle of "like cures like": if a particular substance causes symptoms in a healthy person, it can be used to relieve the same symptoms in a sick person.

Homeopathic remedies are derived mostly from plant, mineral, or animal materials. Homeopaths believe that when a concentrated solution, known as the "mother tincture," is diluted and shaken to make a remedy, it becomes more effective; this process is termed "potentization." It can be argued that, because these solutions are unlikely to contain even one molecule of the original substance, they cannot have any effect. In contrast, homeopaths believe that, somehow, the water molecules preserve a "memory" or "energy" of the substance. They are convinced that this energy is effective. Homeopaths believe that their remedies stimulate the body's own natural healing processes, and they try to treat the whole person rather than just a symptom or disease.

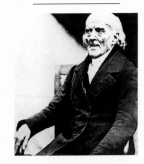

DR. HAHNEMANN

Hahnemann was born in Meissen, Germany. After six years of experiments, he came up with his famous theory of homeopathy – that "like cures like."

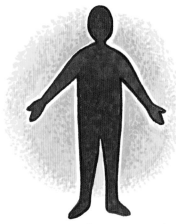

ABOVE *Homeopathy aims at treating the entire body to alleviate illness.*

BELOW *A homeopath prepares remedies in his laboratory.*

DOES IT WORK?

Little scientific investigation has been carried out into homeopathy specifically for the treatment of sleep disorders. There is only one rigorous trial of individualized homeopathic remedies. Its results suggest that patients with insomnia do not benefit more from these medications than from placebos. Since the homeopathic remedies are so dilute they are unlikely to cause serious side effects to the patient. With less dilute remedies, allergies, and other adverse effects are, however, possible.

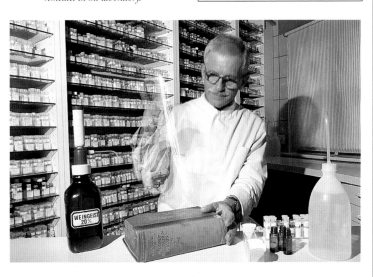

FLOWER REMEDIES

Flower remedies are thought to free energy for self-healing. Flower therapy was developed by Dr. Edward Bach, a British homeopathic physician, in the early part of the 20th century. Bach created 38 remedies and recommended particular flower tinctures for specific emotional problems.

Bach flower remedies are prepared by placing flower petals in spring water and leaving them in the sun for several hours. This process is thought to connect with the flowers' healing energy, which is then conveyed during preparation. From this, tincture is then produced with brandy as a preservative. The remedies are taken by placing drops on the tongue or drinking the tincture with water. Most of the tinctures are made from one species of flower, but the "Rescue Remedy" contains five.

LEFT *Bach flower remedies are prepared using flower petals, water, and brandy.*

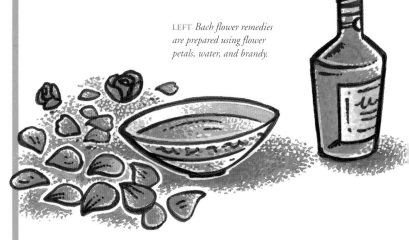

EMOTIONAL LIFT

Flower remedies are thought to lift the emotions; as a result, the body is free to heal itself. Advocates of the therapy believe that a negative emotional state is the underlying cause of most illnesses, and certainly of most cases of insomnia. In contrast, homeopathic

DR. BACH

Welsh-born homeopathic physician Edward Bach experimented on himself when he was developing the flower remedies. "Disease is in the essence the result of conflict between the Soul and the Mind," he said.

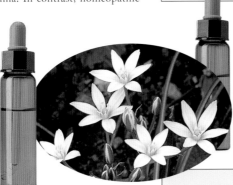
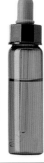

ABOVE *Flower remedies are made from a variety of blooms, including the "Star of Bethlehem".*

Doctor,Bach argued that his remedies helped to prevent mental attitudes from causing physical illness.

Improving the emotional state should help to cure a sleep problem. Therefore, these remedies might have a place in the treatment of insomnia.

DOES IT WORK?

There is no scientific evidence to back up any of the claims for flower remedies, although there are plenty of testimonials of supposed beneficial effects. It is possible that these may be due to placebo effects, e.g. resulting from the expectation that the tinctures would help. Consequently, at present the value of these remedies for treating insomnia is not known.

ACUPUNCTURE

A traditional Chinese treatment, acupuncture involves the
insertion of fine needles to stimulate specific parts of the
body. The aim of the treatment is to create a state of
balanced harmony within the body.

Acupuncture's history goes back for at least 2,000 years. The first textbook called *Huang-di Ni-jing*, or the *Yellow Emperor's Classic of Internal Medicine*, was produced some time between 300 and 100 BC. Acupuncture forms just one component of Traditional Chinese Medicine (TCM), and works in conjunction with herbal medicine, massage, manipulation, relaxation techniques, and diet.

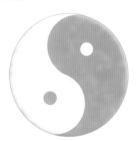

ABOVE Yin *is dark and female, and*
yang *is active, light, and male.*

THE CONCEPT

Traditional acupuncturists believe that energy known as *Qi* (pronounced "che" as in cheese) moves in everything. *Qi* polarizes into the complementary forces of *yin* and *yang*. These forces are in dynamic balance in a healthy person, producing a state of harmony, or *Tao*. *Qi* is thought to flow through the body in invisible pathways called meridians.

Ill health is thought to be a consequence of an imbalance between *yin* and *yang*. The aim is to restore the balance. Acupuncture is seen as one way of achieving this state of energy balance by stimulating points on the meridians to unblock energy if it has become stuck, or to speed it up or slow it down as is necessary.

THE MERIDIANS

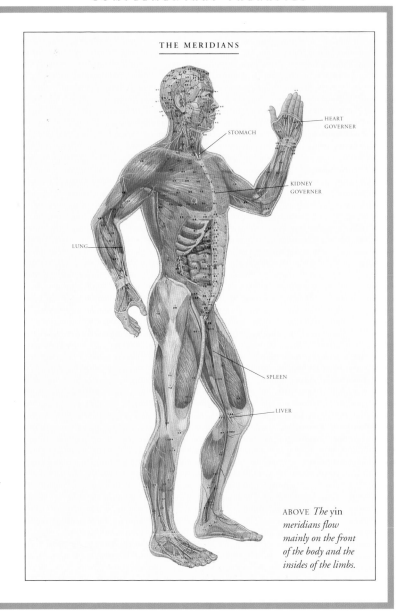

HEART
GOVERNER

STOMACH

KIDNEY
GOVERNER

LUNG

SPLEEN

LIVER

ABOVE *The* yin
*meridians flow
mainly on the front
of the body and the
insides of the limbs.*

WESTERN VIEW

Western acupuncturists are convinced that there are understandable biological mechanisms to explain the effects of acupuncture. It is thought that acupuncture acts by influencing the nervous system, which is responsible for transmitting messages around the body, and to and from the brain. In addition, acupuncture may well stimulate the release of chemical messengers within the nervous system, aptly called neurotransmitters. This could be the way in which it helps relieve insomnia and other illnesses.

ABOVE *A variety of different needles are used according to the treatment.*

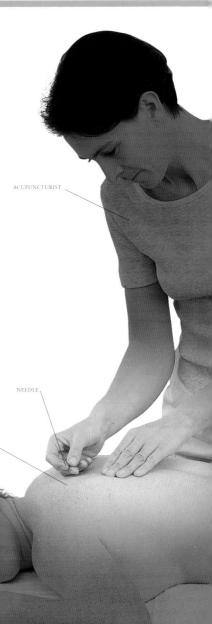

ACUPUNCTURIST

NEEDLE

POINT ON MERIDIAN

PATIENT

DOES IT WORK?

Few clinical trials have been carried out to test whether acupuncture enhances sleep. Certainly no conclusive rigorous studies exist so far. At present, we simply cannot tell whether acupuncture is helpful for insomnia, or little more than a placebo, but it is well worth a try.

LEFT *Having diagnosed the patient, the acupuncturist determines to treat the* yang *meridians which flow mainly on the back.*

IS IT SAFE?

Like any intervention, acupuncture is not totally risk free. Bruising, fainting, and local skin infections occur frequently. Serious complications, such as puncturing a lung (*pneumothorax*) or heart (*cardiac tamponade*), are much rarer. Needling should be avoided in people with a bleeding disorder or taking blood-thinning medications. Those who rely on a cardiac pacemaker should not use electroacupuncture. Good practitioners will sterilize their needles properly or use disposable needles to avoid the risk of transmitting infections such as hepatitis and HIV. In several countries there is no law to stop anyone from setting themselves up as an acupuncturist. It is therefore necessary to ensure that a practitioner is properly qualified (see pages 80–81).

EXERCISE

Exercise and physical activity are associated with a feeling of well-being. It has been suggested that exercise might act in a variety of different ways to enhance sleep.

One of the ways exercise can help insomnia is to provide a distraction from unhappy thoughts that otherwise might obstruct sleep. Most obviously perhaps, physical activity wears you out and this brings tiredness and good sleep. Exercise can improve the fitness and efficiency of the heart and lungs, and help to reduce the symptoms of tension and anxiety. Exercise may also stimulate the body to produce chemicals called endorphins that relieve pain, raise mood, and increase well-being. When done correctly, exercise is very safe and carries only few health risks. Therefore, it is well worth considering as part of a comprehensive strategy for enhancing sleep.

THE BEST FORM

Walking, dancing, running, cycling, swimming, and team sports such as football and hockey are typical "aerobic" exercises. This means that they involve physical work sustained over relatively long periods, which improves the efficiency of the heart and lungs. So called "anaerobic" exercises involve high intensity work for very short periods, as in

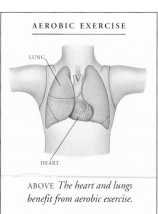

AEROBIC EXERCISE

LUNG

HEART

ABOVE *The heart and lungs benefit from aerobic exercise.*

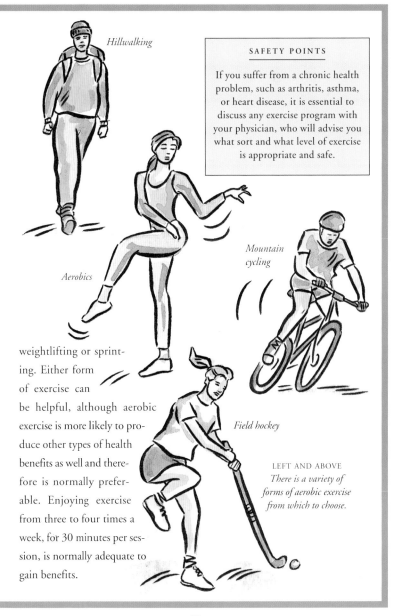

Hillwalking

SAFETY POINTS

If you suffer from a chronic health problem, such as arthritis, asthma, or heart disease, it is essential to discuss any exercise program with your physician, who will advise you what sort and what level of exercise is appropriate and safe.

Mountain cycling

Aerobics

weightlifting or sprinting. Either form of exercise can be helpful, although aerobic exercise is more likely to produce other types of health benefits as well and therefore is normally preferable. Enjoying exercise from three to four times a week, for 30 minutes per session, is normally adequate to gain benefits.

Field hockey

LEFT AND ABOVE
There is a variety of forms of aerobic exercise from which to choose.

59

HYPNOTHERAPY

Under hypnosis a trance is induced that makes the person
deeply relaxed, allowing him or her to be receptive to
suggestions made by the therapist.

Although in an altered state of consciousness, hypnotized people are aware of what is happening around them and can hear what is being said. Hypnotherapists assure us that people cannot be made to do anything against their will when they are hypnotized.

Hypnotherapists believe that they can produce rapid results by directly influencing the unconscious mind.

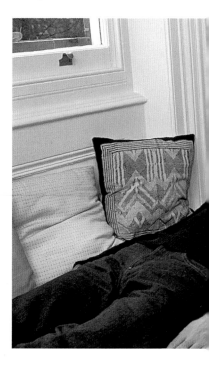

THE POWER
OF SUGGESTION

Most people can be hypnotized if they want to be. Clients can be guided into a hypnotized state by the use of relaxation methods, imagery, and visualization techniques. The therapist may make suggestions aimed at changing the way the client experiences or responds to something. For example, the therapist may suggest that the client will no longer feel anxious.

FALSE MEMORY

Sometimes hypnosis can create unpleasant false memories. These often make headlines under the term "false memory syndrome" and have been known to ruin peoples' lives. Care should therefore be taken to avoid the possibility of an unscrupulous practitioner taking advantage of someone who is vulnerable.

DOES IT WORK?

So far there is little scientific evidence that hypnosis can be helpful for sleep problems. Yet it is quite clear that hypnotherapy can enhance relaxation and reduce anxiety. If insomnia is related to anxiety or inner tension, which it is in many instances, hypnotherapy might be helpful.

BELOW *Hypnotherapists claim they can directly influence the unconscious mind.*

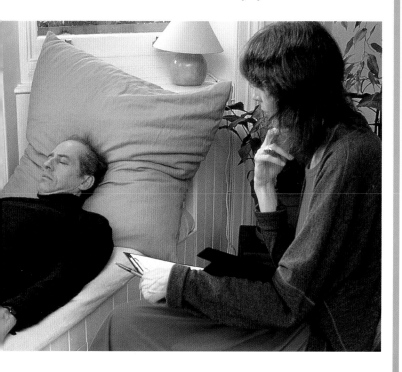

AUTOGENIC TRAINING

This technique of autosuggestion was developed in Germany and is relatively unknown in English-speaking countries. It might be of considerable benefit for people suffering from sleep disturbances.

Autogenic training is normally taught in small groups by a certified teacher. The group participants usually lie on the floor and are taught, through simple exercises, to experience certain basic sensations.

The group participant will mentally repeat these messages and, in turn, actually experience these sensations. Once these first lessons have been mastered, more complicated tasks ensue. The participant will, for instance, be taught to control the body's autonomic function, e.g. to slow heart rate. Foremost, one learns how to achieve almost total relaxation of body and mind.

TYPICAL
SENSATION EXAMPLES

Simple exercises can help us to regulate complex body functions:

✧ My left foot becomes heavy.

✧ My left foot becomes warm.

✧ My left foot becomes warm and heavy.

RIGHT *Autogenic training is best given to small groups of people.*

THE ROUTINE

Classes are normally held once a week. After about eight classes and regular home practice, you are usually able to carry out these exercises without further supervision. It is important that the exercises are performed on a regular, ideally daily, basis.

WILL IT HELP?

There are only a few controlled trials of autogenic training. Those relating to insomnia suggest that it is a useful method to improve sleep. By learning to control breathing and body temperature, you increase the possibility of being able to relax and drop off to sleep. The technique is almost entirely free of side effects. Moreover it is not expensive. Autogenic training is therefore recommended for people suffering from insomnia as an attempt to enhance sleep.

HEALING

Spiritual or faith healing, whereby energy is channeled into a patient to help a complaint – often through the "laying on of hands" – is a popular way to treat insomnia.

Healing, usually referred to as spiritual or faith healing, is an ancient form of treatment in which practitioners are regarded as having the "gift" to cure. Stories of the healing power date back to the time of Jesus, and in the *New Testament* (1 Corinthians 12:9) healing is listed among the rewards bestowed on the faithful. During the Middle Ages, it was believed that kings and saints were blessed with the power to heal.

Today, healing, through a technique termed as the "laying on of hands," is a widespread practice, not limited just to the Christian belief. In the UK, healers form the largest group of complementary practitioners.

TRANSMITTING ENERGY

Healers claim they can link up to an undefinable source of "energy" – this may be referred to as God. This energy is thought to be transmitted to the patient, and the complaint cures itself. The healer has no active powers but is a mere instrument for channeling the energy. According to healers, most health problems are amenable to healing, insomnia included.

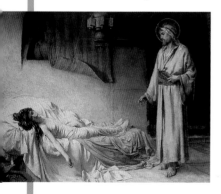

LEFT *Healing has been practiced for centuries and is part of the Christian faith.*

HEALER TRANSMITS
ENERGY TO CURE
HER PATIENT

"LAYING ON
OF HANDS"

HEALING HANDS

During a healing session, the patient is normally asked to sit or lie quietly while the healer moves his or her hands over the body, locates areas of malfunction, and transmits the healing energy. Many patients experience a sensation of warmth under the healing hands. A session lasts about 30 minutes and patients often feel refreshed and relaxed afterward.

LEFT *A healer "lays on hands" without actually touching her patient.*

DOES IT WORK?

From the few controlled studies of healing that have been carried out, there is a suggestion that healing can produce an effect. Most trials are, however, burdened with methodological problems. No study of healing for insomnia has been published, so its value for sleep disorders is impossible to judge. If done properly and with the knowledge of your doctor, it may be worth trying as a way of relieving symptoms.

TAI CHI

A routine of gentle and relaxing exercises originating in China, Tai Chi is believed to improve well-being. To this effect it may help those with sleeping difficulties.

Tai Chi is an ancient form of Chinese exercise, involving a program of controlled slow movements, meditation, concentration, and breathing exercises. It is still practiced

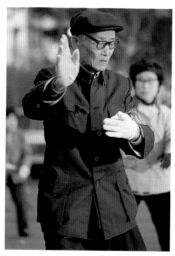

ABOVE *Tai Chi has been practiced in China for millennia. It is a graceful, invigorating form of exercise.*

> ### DOES IT WORK?
>
> In the past few years, since its rise in popularity in the West, Tai Chi has been investigated scientifically. Results of several clinical trials suggest that it does indeed convey health benefits, particularly in the elderly. Whilst there have been no trials specifically related to insomnia, the relaxing effects of Tai Chi may well help people who suffer from sleeping difficulties.

in China on a daily basis by millions of people, particularly by the elderly, and is becoming very popular in the West as a health-promoting activity.

The aim of Tai Chi is to build up strength, create rhythm and balance your body's inert energy. Traditionally it has strong links with acupuncture.

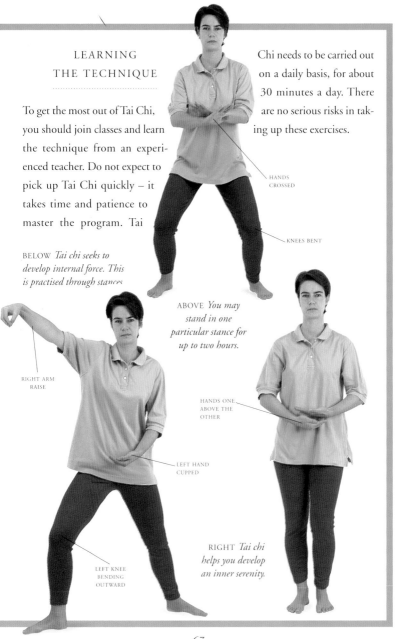

LEARNING THE TECHNIQUE

To get the most out of Tai Chi, you should join classes and learn the technique from an experienced teacher. Do not expect to pick up Tai Chi quickly – it takes time and patience to master the program. Tai

Chi needs to be carried out on a daily basis, for about 30 minutes a day. There are no serious risks in taking up these exercises.

HANDS CROSSED

KNEES BENT

BELOW *Tai chi seeks to develop internal force. This is practised through stances*

ABOVE *You may stand in one particular stance for up to two hours.*

RIGHT ARM RAISE

HANDS ONE ABOVE THE OTHER

LEFT HAND CUPPED

LEFT KNEE BENDING OUTWARD

RIGHT *Tai chi helps you develop an inner serenity.*

REFLEXOLOGY

Reflexologists believe that deep massage on certain parts of the feet can correct disorders within the body.

Reflexologists base their work on the principle that the inner organs and parts of the body are represented on the sole of the foot in the form of "reflex zones." Maps of the feet have been drawn up by reflexologists to show the zones and their connected body parts.

WHAT HAPPENS DURING THERAPY?

First, a therapist massages the foot in order to find resistance or the impression of crystals in the subcutaneous tissues of the sole, since this is believed to indicate a problem. When resistance is identified, the therapist locates the malfunction within the body by referring to the map of reflex zones. Following this diagnostic step, the therapist then treats the abnormalities found by applying deep mas-

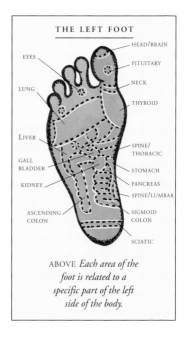

THE LEFT FOOT

HEAD/BRAIN
EYES
PITUITARY
NECK
LUNG
THYROID
LIVER
SPINE/THORACIC
GALL BLADDER
STOMACH
KIDNEY
PANCREAS
SPINE/LUMBAR
ASCENDING COLON
SIGMOID COLON
SCIATIC

ABOVE *Each area of the foot is related to a specific part of the left side of the body.*

sage to the relative zone on the sole of the foot. Reflexologists believe that as the massage dissolves the resistance in the tissue, so the malfunction of the body disappears.

The intensity of the massage on the foot can cause a certain amount of pain, but most people experience the treatment as relaxing and pleasurable. A typical session is normally about 20 minutes long.

DOES REFLEXOLOGY WORK?

To date no trial on reflexology as a treatment for insomnia has been published. Therefore, it is not easy to give advice. There is certainly little scope for harm. There is also little doubt that reflexology can be a most relaxing experience. Consequently, if you can afford it, the therapy may be worth a try.

HOW EFFECTIVE IS THE TREATMENT?

There is little rigorous research into the area of reflexology. Investigations indicate that as a diagnostic tool reflexology is not reliable. First, the diagnoses achieved do not correspond to diagnoses validated by doctors. Second, they differ almost at random among a group of well-trained reflexologists. Several clinical trials of reflexology as a therapy exist, some with positive, others with negative, results.

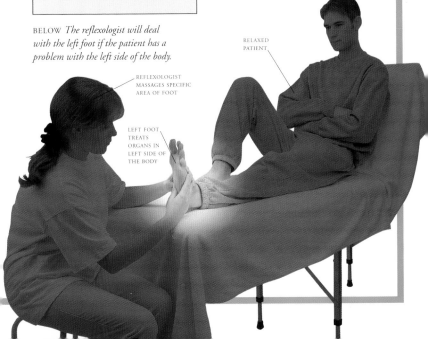

BELOW *The reflexologist will deal with the left foot if the patient has a problem with the left side of the body.*

RELAXED PATIENT

REFLEXOLOGIST MASSAGES SPECIFIC AREA OF FOOT

LEFT FOOT TREATS ORGANS IN LEFT SIDE OF THE BODY

MASSAGE THERAPY

Massage is a well-established way of relaxing the muscles
and the mind. A soothing experience, massage can help
to encourage sleep.

Many different massage techniques exist. They consist of a range of manual manipulative techniques on the muscles and soft tissues of the body. The therapist employs a variety of kneading, rubbing, pressing, and stretching movements. These improve the blood flow, relax muscles, and quiet the mind. The intensity of massage can vary from soft and agreeable to vigorous and uncomfortable.

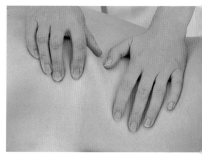

ABOVE *Massage helps to relax and detoxify the body.*

DIFFERENT APPROACHES

Massage is one of the oldest forms of treatment known to mankind, and various types of massage are found within all the major medical traditions of the world. The classical "Western" massage, which has seen a recent revival in the United States and the UK, focuses on toning the muscles; this technique originated in Sweden. An Oriental style of massage, known as Shiatsu, is derived from acupuncture and aims to clear "energy blockages" through massage of the acupuncture points, while from India, marma massage is used as part of Ayurvedic medicine and is a very brisk technique used to stimulate specific points on the body.

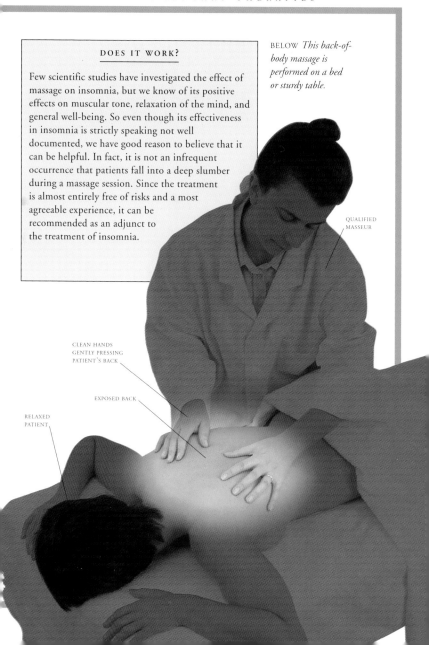

DOES IT WORK?

Few scientific studies have investigated the effect of massage on insomnia, but we know of its positive effects on muscular tone, relaxation of the mind, and general well-being. So even though its effectiveness in insomnia is strictly speaking not well documented, we have good reason to believe that it can be helpful. In fact, it is not an infrequent occurrence that patients fall into a deep slumber during a massage session. Since the treatment is almost entirely free of risks and a most agreeable experience, it can be recommended as an adjunct to the treatment of insomnia.

BELOW *This back-of-body massage is performed on a bed or sturdy table.*

QUALIFIED MASSEUR

CLEAN HANDS GENTLY PRESSING PATIENT'S BACK

EXPOSED BACK

RELAXED PATIENT

AROMATHERAPY

Aromatherapy involves the use of essential oils, which have therapeutic qualities, to heal the body and relax the mind. Generally the oils are massaged into the skin, although they can also be inhaled, used in the bath, or applied as a cold compress.

The essential oils employed in aromatherapy are extracted from the flowers, fruit, seeds, leaves, and roots of plants. An aromatherapist selects the oils according to the physical and emotional state of the client. The selected oils may be blended together and are generally massaged (immersed in a carrier oil) into the skin to produce the desired effects. Adding the essential oils to a bath is an easy way of appreciating the effects of aromatherapy at home. It is thought that each oil has specific qualities, for example that lavender oil is calming and sleep-inducing.

BELOW *Aromatherapy oils should be heated for effective dispersal, but you can add them to baths or even soap.*

OIL DISPERSED BY HEAT FROM CANDLE

DOES IT WORK?

Scientifically, it is still not known whether the oils themselves, or the method of application, or even the combination of both, are responsible for the perceived effects. But undoubtedly, many people who have tried the therapy believe that it is relaxing, reduces anxiety, and generally helps them to feel better. This is also borne out by two clinical trials. In these studies, patients with sleep problems were given lavender oil to inhale. Even though the trials are burdened with several flaws, their results suggest that lavender oil improved the quality of daytime wakefulness and led to a more sustained sleep.

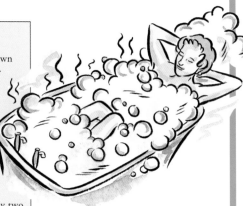

ABOVE *Always mix essential oils with a base oil before applying them to the skin.*

CAUTION!

Essential oils are powerful mixtures of plant chemicals. They are on unrestricted sale in the United States and the UK, often without any instructions. They should not be applied directly to the skin or taken orally in undiluted form. It is important to be aware that some oils, such as orange, lemon, or bergamot, can sensitize the skin to sunlight so burning can occur much more easily. Some oils are known to promote cancerous growths in laboratory tests, but there is no evidence that this also occurs in humans. Because the skin absorbs the chemicals from the oils, they are best avoided in pregnancy.

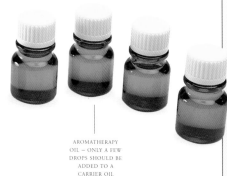

AROMATHERAPY OIL – ONLY A FEW DROPS SHOULD BE ADDED TO A CARRIER OIL

MUSIC THERAPY

Music can be used therapeutically to arouse positive and calming feelings within us. Its relaxing influence can also play a role in curing insomnia.

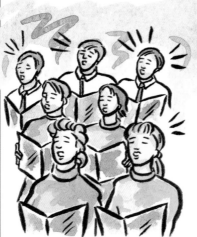

LEFT *Singing promotes good health and happiness.*

individual or in a group setting. The music therapist assesses the patient and then selects appropriate music for the condition, often with a great deal of input from the patient. Music may help to provide a distraction from present circumstances and aid the recall of pleasant associations from the past.

The belief behind music therapy is that we all have the inborn ability to respond to music. Indeed, for many people particular pieces of music are associated with certain events and feelings in their lives.

There are several forms of music therapy; they may involve listening to music, singing or playing music as an

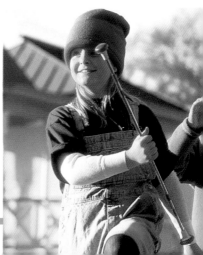

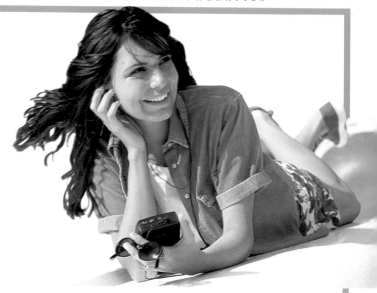

ABOVE *It is possible to listen to music almost anywhere you go; try combining fresh air and your favorite piece.*

DOES IT WORK?

Many reports about the benefits of music therapy are anecdotal, but there are a few interesting results from the small number of scientific investigations that have been carried out. Most of the studies do not involve the treatment of insomnia. Therefore, it is difficult to judge the place of music therapy in treating sleep disorders. Yet we all know that listening to certain pieces of music can be intensely relaxing. We should use such experiences wisely when we want to promote sleep.

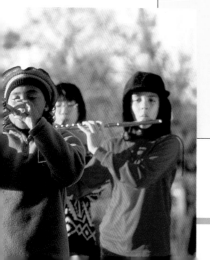

LEFT *Anyone can join in a music ensemble, even if they only get to bang a drum.*

YOGA

Based on ancient Hindu philosophy, yoga comprises
a set of disciplined exercises, combined with relaxation
and breathing techniques. It is widely recognized
in the West for having beneficial effects
on health.

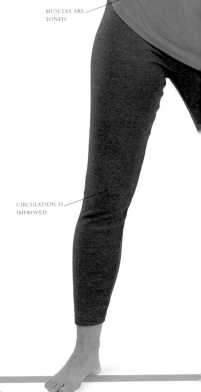

A highly disciplined activity, yoga
promotes fitness, flexibility of
movement, relaxation, and general
well-being.

MUSCLES ARE
TONED

A LIFESTYLE

To master the techniques involved in
yoga, you will need to learn from an
experienced teacher, either in a group
or on an individual basis. The way to
derive the maximum benefit from the
discipline is to make it a regular part
of your life. Practice on a weekly or
even daily basis will maintain general
flexibility and reduce tension. As you
become more accustomed to the prac-
tise of yoga, you will find that it
becomes more and more beneficial.

CIRCULATION IS
IMPROVED

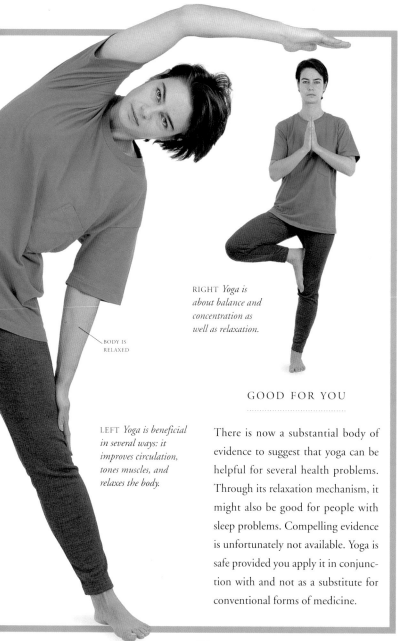

RIGHT *Yoga is about balance and concentration as well as relaxation.*

BODY IS RELAXED

LEFT *Yoga is beneficial in several ways: it improves circulation, tones muscles, and relaxes the body.*

GOOD FOR YOU

There is now a substantial body of evidence to suggest that yoga can be helpful for several health problems. Through its relaxation mechanism, it might also be good for people with sleep problems. Compelling evidence is unfortunately not available. Yoga is safe provided you apply it in conjunction with and not as a substitute for conventional forms of medicine.

RELAXATION THERAPIES

Most complementary therapies include an element of relaxation. In addition, a number of specific relaxation methods are available; they all aim to decrease inner tension, which has a place in helping insomnia.

The aims of relaxation therapies can be to slow breathing, reduce heart rate, and lower muscle tension. Relaxation classes may be available through adult education services, health centers, or sports centers. Audiotapes can be bought that guide you through the relaxation process. Undoubtedly, a relaxed body and mind will help you to sleep better – the following exercise is worth trying.

RELAXATION EXERCISE

Lie down on a mat on the floor, close your eyes and start to breathe slowly as if in sleep. Let your arms fall out away from your body, with the palms facing upward, and let your legs fall slightly apart. Tense for a few seconds and then relax each group of muscles in turn, perhaps starting at the feet, and working up the legs and trunk to the arms, neck, and face. In this way the whole body becomes progressively relaxed. Breathe in as you tense the muscles and then breathe out slowly and allow your muscles to relax.

FEET FALLING
TO EITHER
SIDE

Meanwhile, think of a pleasant peaceful setting, such as lying on a sunny beach. Once the whole body is relaxed, allow yourself to remain in that state for five or ten minutes, breathing regularly, slowly, and deeply.

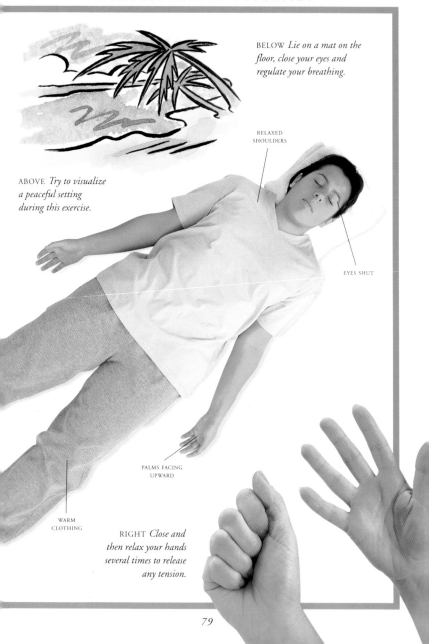

BELOW *Lie on a mat on the floor, close your eyes and regulate your breathing.*

RELAXED SHOULDERS

ABOVE *Try to visualize a peaceful setting during this exercise.*

EYES SHUT

PALMS FACING UPWARD

WARM CLOTHING

RIGHT *Close and then relax your hands several times to release any tension.*

CHOOSING A COMPLEMENTARY THERAPIST

Here we give you guidance on how to go about finding the right therapist for your needs.

Since complementary medicine is largely unregulated, finding a competent and experienced therapist can be a minefield. Unquestionably, there are many highly qualified complementary practitioners but there are also less-qualified ones and even outright charlatans. Once you have made up your mind to try a certain complementary therapy, you must be careful to choose a well-trained and responsible professional.

One of the best ways to find a reliable practitioner is to follow a recommendation from your doctor. Many doctors have now become open-minded and have established good working relationships with complementary practitioners. If this is not possible, try to get a recommendation from someone you trust and who you know is critical. Make sure your practitioner is not just starting in the profession – check that he or she has had several years training, and belongs to a reputable professional organization. He or she should have indemnity cover.

RIGHT *Always research the history of your practitioner.*

PRACTITIONERS CHECKLIST

At your first visit, it is essential that you ask the practitioner the following questions, so that you can be sure that you are making the right choice.

If the practitioner refuses to answer any or some of these questions, or if the answers do not completely satisfy you, change your therapist.

Remember to ask
- What qualifications do you have?
- How long have you practised?
- Which professional body do you belong to?
- Have you got insurance cover?
- Do you think that you can cure my insomnia?
- What exactly does the therapy involve?
- What side effects may occur?
- How many treatment sessions will be required?
- How much will it cost?

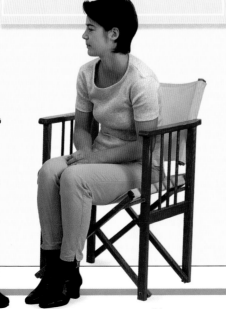

BEWARE OF THERAPISTS WHO:

❖

Interfere with your physician's prescriptions.

❖

Promise a quick and total cure. (If it sounds too good to be true, it usually is!)

❖

Claim that their method of treatment is the only one that can help you.

❖

Speak badly about other healthcare professionals.

❖

Claim that their method is entirely free of risks.

❖

Boast of suspicious-looking qualifications that cannot be scrutinized.

COMBINING TREATMENTS

A multifactorial approach is best for insomnia since it is a multifactorial problem. Many complementary therapies can be combined in a meaningful way. You may, for instance, use herbal, massage, and exercise treatments in parallel. But do try to avoid using conventional sleeping pills and herbal treatments in parallel without expert supervision.

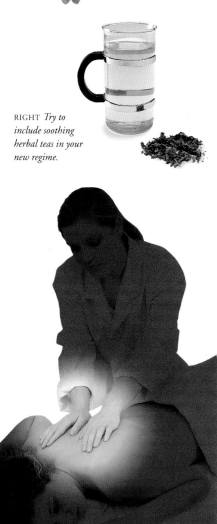

RIGHT *Try to include soothing herbal teas in your new regime.*

Otherwise, it makes a lot of sense to combine the best of the "two worlds" of complementary and mainstream medicine. You should, of course, always see your physician when you have insomnia. Discuss the options with him or her and follow prescriptions and advice. Tell your physician which complementary therapies you use in addition to the treatment he or she advises. You should also report to him or her any therapeutic success or failure of the treatments you have tried.

RIGHT *Many people find that massage is a successful alternative therapy.*

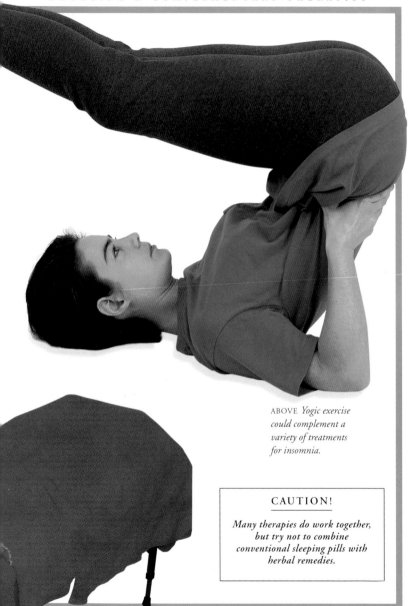

ABOVE *Yogic exercise could complement a variety of treatments for insomnia.*

CAUTION!

Many therapies do work together, but try not to combine conventional sleeping pills with herbal remedies.

PRACTICAL TIPS FOR PEOPLE WITH SLEEP PROBLEMS

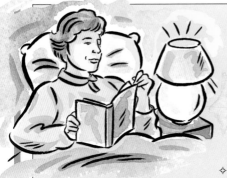

ABOVE *A regular routine will help you overcome insomnia.*

✧ Maintain your usual schedule of wake and sleep and avoid irregularity as much as you can.

✧ Avoid stimulants such as tobacco, alcohol, tea, or coffee in the evening and late afternoon.

✧ Make sure you have enough exercise several hours before going to bed so that you are physically tired at bedtime.

✧ Don't go to bed before it is really time to sleep, and use your bedroom only for sleep (and sex).

✧ Don't try to force yourself to fall asleep; it won't work.

✧ If you can't sleep, do something to distract you, e.g. read a book.

✧ Avoid worrying while waiting to fall asleep.

✧ Talk worries over well before bedtime, so that you have them "out of your system."

✧ Consider taking a hot bath before going to sleep.

✧ Consider taking a sauna in the afternoon.

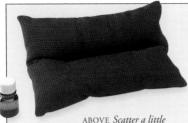

ABOVE *Scatter a little lavender oil on your pillow before you go to bed.*

✧ Observe yourself and you may find out exactly which eating habits are best for your sleep.

✧ Go to the lavatory before you go to bed.

✧ Make sure your room is neither too hot nor too cold.

✧ Try scenting the bedroom with lavender oil.

✧ If possible, make sure no noise will disturb your sleep.

✧ Try a lavender-filled cushion.

✧ Avoid an irregular lifestyle in every sense.

✧ Use music for relaxation before bedtime.

✧ If you sleep badly for a while, don't panic – it's normal and not dangerous!

✧ If you wake up at night with your head full of ideas, write them down. It will allow you to forget about them and make it easier to fall back to sleep.

✧ If you snore and are overweight, reduce your weight and avoid alcohol.

✧ If you sleep badly at night, do not take naps during the day.

RIGHT *Exercise is bound to help insomnia, simply because a tired body creates a sleepy mind.*

✧ Avoid heavy meals in the evening; eat several hours before bedtime.

MANAGING INSOMNIA

Everyone must learn to accept periods of insomnia.
It affects the concentration the following day and is
depressing, but remember: insomnia doesn't make you
ill and nobody ever died of it.

Twelve steps for a good night's sleep:

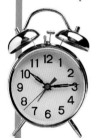

1 *Bedtime must be regular – within 30 minutes of the same time each day.*

2 *Don't lie in bed in the morning: rise as soon as you wake.*

3 *Avoid sleeping during the day, but take some exercise instead.*

4 *Establish a regular routine before bed: a gentle stroll with the dog; or making a milk drink will do, and the warm drink might be comforting too.*

5 *Do not use stimulants for at least an hour before bed: this includes coffee and alcohol, and (smokers) means cutting down on cigarettes for this hour.*

6 *Make sure you are not hungry – but neither should your stomach be uncomfortably full.*

7 *Control your thoughts: Do not do any work for at least an hour before bed – similarly do not try to sort out any ongoing problems or worries. Put pen and paper beside your bed, then you can catch any brainwaves you get during the night. On the other hand, if you have any guilty feelings or resentments hanging over from the day, then think of them positively, try to accept the situation, and be reassured that you're not unique in this!*

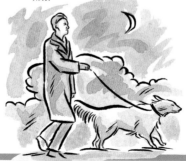

8 When you get into bed, make sure your position is comfortable and the room temperature is normal.

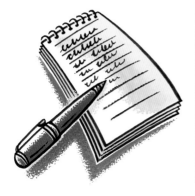

9 Many people find that reading a light novel for 10 minutes is relaxing (nothing too stimulating or worrying!).

10 You may want to play soft music with a snooze switch set for 30 minutes.

11 Once you switch off the light and get comfortable, you are only allowed to move once! Moving around and fidgeting keeps you awake.

12 Take two deep, slow breaths and perform the relaxation exercise four times. By the time you reach the head you are usually asleep.

IF YOU WAKE UP

Figure out what woke you up and deal with it. If your bladder is full then go to the toilet – but do not make a habit of this. Your worries are bound to come to your attention before long; go back to number 12. Above all don't let your body start to fidget – you must not move! When you get the urge to move, really concentrate on resisting it, make it your sole purpose. With any luck, the next thing you know is it's morning and time to get up.

SLEEPING TABLETS

Don't be tempted by sleeping tablets except when it is crucial that you get some sleep; even then, don't take them for more than three nights in a row, so that you don't become dependent on them.

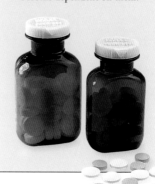

FURTHER READING

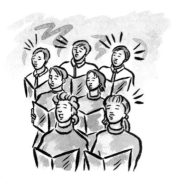

Ball, N., and Hough, N.
The Sleep Solution
(Vermilion, 1998)

Cassileth, B.R.
The Alternative Medicine Handbook
(Norton WW, USA, 1998)

Corrigan, D.
*Herbal Medicine for
Sleep and Relaxation*
(Amberwood Publishing, 1996)

Digeronimo, T.
Insomnia: 50 Essential Things to Do
(Plume, 1997)

Ernst, E. (ed.)
The Book of Symptoms and Treatments
(Element, 1998)

Fugh-Berman, A.
Alternative Medicine: What Works?
(Odonian Press, USA, 1996)

Guilleminault, C.
Sleep and its Disorders in Children
(Raven Press, 1987)

Hoffmann, D.
*Herbs for a Good Night's Sleep: Herbal
Approaches to Relieving Insomnia
Safely and Effectively.
Understand your Sleeplessness –
and Banish it Forever!*
(Keats Publications, 1997)

Inlander, C.B., and Moran, C.K.
67 Ways to Good Sleep
(Random House, 1998)

Johnson, T.S., and Halberstadt, J.
*Phantom of the Night, Overcome
Sleep Apnea Syndrome and Snoring –
Win Your Hidden Struggling to
Breathe, Sleep and Live*
(New Technology Publishing, 1992)

Keane, C. (ed.)
The Stress File
(Blackwater Press, 1997)

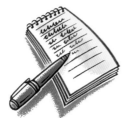

Kermani, K.
Autogenic Training: Effective Holistic Way to Better Health
(Souvenir Press, 1996)

Lavery, S.
The Healthing Power of Sleep: How to Achieve Restorative Sleep Naturally
(Firesdie, 1997)

Lipman, D.S.
Snoring from A to Zzz: Proven Cures for the Night's Worst Nuisance
(Spencer Press, 1997)

Maxwell-Hudson, C.
The Complete Book of Massage
(Doring Kindersley, 1998)

Morgan, D.R.
Sleep Secrets for Shiftworkers & People with Off-Beat Schedules
(Whole Person Associates, 1996)

O'Hanlon, B.
Sleep. The Common Sense Approach
(Newleaf, 1998)

Pascualy, R.A., and Soest, S.W.
Snoring and Sleep Apnea. Personal and Family Guide to Diagnosis and Treatment
(Demos Vermande, 1996)

Price, S.
Aromatherapy for Common Ailments
(Gaia Books, 1991)

Scott, E.
The Natural Way to Sound Sleep
(Orion Books, 1996)

Vickers, A.
Massage and Aromatherapy
(Chapman Hall, 1996)

Weekes, C.
Self Help for Your Nerves
(Thorsons, 1995)

Wilson, V.N.
Sleep Thief, Restless Legs Syndrome
(Galaxy Books, 1996)

USEFUL ADDRESSES

**American Association of Acupuncture
and Oriental Medicine**
1400 16th Street NW
Washington DC 20036 USA

American Counselling Association
5999 Stevenson Avenue
Alexandria, VA 22304-330 USA

American Yoga Association
513 S Orange Avenue
Satasota, FL 34236 USA

**Association of Medical
Aromatherapists**
11 Park Circus
Glasgow G3 6AX

Association of Reflexologists
27 Old Gloucester Street
London WC1N 3XX UK

**British Association
for Counselling**
37a Sheep Street
Rugby
Warwickshire CV21 3BX UK

**British Herbal
Medicine Association**
Sun House
Church Street
Stroud
Gloucestershire GL5 1JL UK

Dr Edward Bach Foundation
Mount Vernon
Bakers Lane
Sarwell
Oxon OX10 0PZ UK

Homeopathic Educational Services
2124 Kittredge Street
Berkeley, CA 94704 USA

**Institute for Music, Health
and Education**
PO Box 4179
Boulder, CO 80306 USA

Iyengar Yoga
2404 27th Avenue
San Francisco, CA 94116 USA

**National Association of
Music Therapy**
1500 Massachusettes Avenue NW
Suite 42
Silver Springs, MD 20910 USA

National Center for Homeopathy
801 North Fairfax Street
Suite 396
Alexandria, VA 22314 USA

Sleep Apnea Clinic
St Vincen's Hospital
Elm Park
Dublin 4 IRELAND

INDEX

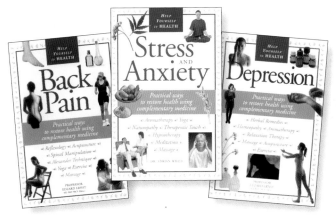

Picture Acknowledgements

a=above; b=below; r=right